Diabetes

How to Effectively Lower Your Blood Sugar Without Medication Using Natural Remedies and Recipes

Robert S. Lee

Contents

Chapter 1. The Importance of Controlling Diabetes...........11

Chapter 2. Smoothie Recipes to Help Out...... 21

Chapter 3. Herbal Remedies for Quick Control 40

Chapter 4. Dinner Recipes That Will Work.... 55

Chapter 5. Snacks & A Few Extra Recipes...... 77

Chapter 6. Herbal Teas That Produce Results 95

Chapter 7. Herbal Supplements for Strong Results.. 111

Chapter 8. Some Bonus Recipes to Try......... 124

© **Copyright 2019 by Robert S. Lee- All rights reserved.**

This document is geared toward providing exact and reliable information in regard to the topic and issue covered. The publication is sold with the idea that the publisher is not required to render accounting, officially permitted, or otherwise, qualified services. If advice is necessary, legal or professional, a practiced individual in the profession should be ordered.

- From a Declaration of Principles which was accepted and approved equally by a Committee of the American Bar Association and a Committee of Publishers and Associations.

In no way is it legal to reproduce, duplicate, or transmit any part of this document in either electronic means or in printed format. Recording of this publication is strictly prohibited and any storage of this document is not allowed unless with written permission from the publisher. All rights reserved.

The information provided herein is stated to be truthful and consistent, in that any liability, in terms of inattention or otherwise, by any usage or abuse of any policies, processes, or directions contained within is the solitary and utter responsibility of the recipient reader. Under no circumstances will any legal responsibility or blame be held against the publisher for any reparation, damages, or monetary loss due to the information herein, either directly or indirectly.

Respective authors own all copyrights not held by the publisher.

The information herein is offered for informational purposes solely, and is universal as so. The presentation of the information is without contract or any type of guarantee assurance.

The trademarks that are used are without any consent, and the publication of the trademark is without permission or backing by the trademark owner. All trademarks and brands within this book are for clarifying purposes only and are the owned by the owners themselves, not affiliated with this document.

Chapter 1. The Importance of Controlling Diabetes

Many people now suffer with diabetes, both type one and type two. Diabetes is actually a group of diseases that mean you have too much sugar in your blood, or it could mean that you have high blood glucose. This is because it is a metabolic disease that stops your body from producing enough insulin, if any, which is what results in this raise in blood glucose. Diabetes doesn't pick just one type of person, and it can strike anyone. It doesn't matter your lifestyle.

It won't make you immune, but there are lifestyle choices that you can pick that will make sure that your chances of becoming a diabetic decrease, and there are lifestyle choices that you make so that you can control your diabetes even if you couldn't prevent it. Millions of people worldwide are affected, and sometimes the best way to control diabetes is the natural way.

From your drinks to your daily routine, you can control your diabetes naturally, decreasing or eliminating your need for prescription medications. Herbal remedies are an especially popular way to control your diabetes and get your life back in your control.

Controlling It Naturally:

Controlling your diabetes naturally can be done for either type one or type two, but if you are looking to eliminate the use of prescription medication, you have to catch it early. Type two diabetes is considered to be less severe because the fluctuation in blood glucose is not as rapid. It is easier to control type two diabetes, but both can be affected and controlled in natural manners. However, with type one, you may need the help of prescription medication along with natural habits, but this can happen with type two as well.

You commonly control diabetes naturally through what you eat, but you can use other herbal remedies such as drinks as well. A proper lifestyle with proper diet and exercise is also important in taking that step to handling your diabetes and controlling your life. There is no reason to feel helpless when there are so many natural paths that you can take to make sure that diabetes doesn't rule your life anymore.

Why Control It:

When you are diagnosed with diabetes, one or two, you may feel like your life is spiraling out of control, and that is one of the main reasons you need to take control back. However, you also need to control your diabetes so that it doesn't ruin your overall health. If you have diabetes, you're at a higher risk for many serious health conditions. However, with the proper lifestyle and treatment, you'll be able to delay or even prevent these complications. From eye complications to neuropathy to sin complications, diabetes can affect ever part of your life. You need to stay alert to any skin complications, such as skin infections or skin disorders. If you have diabetes, these conditions are much more common.

Eye complications are also an issue because those with diabetes are at a higher risk of cataracts and glaucoma, as well as other eye problems. Regular checkups as well as a healthy lifestyle and natural remedies can lower your risk. Neuropathy is yet another serious condition that those with diabetes needs to be on the lookout for, and it's actually nerve damage resulting from your diabetes. About half of the people suffering from diabetes will suffer from nerve damage from light to severe.

Those with diabetes also have a higher risk of high blood pressure, kidney disease, stroke, gastroparesis, and ketones. Diabetes can even cause sexual problems, and it can cause bladder symptoms as well. Both men and women living with diabetes can have sexual problems, including damage to the nerves and small blood vessels in the area, which is the leading cause of issues that develop thereafter. Sexual dysfunction can be experienced due to the damage of the blood vessels in the area. Men can even experience retrograde ejaculation, which is where most of the man's semen if not all of it will go into the bladder instead of outside of the body.

For women suffering from diabetes, they may notice a decrease in vaginal lubrication, which will result in vaginal dryness. It can also cause painful or uncomfortable intercourse and a decreased libido and sexual response. Which can mean that you cannot become aroused or you may no longer be able to remain aroused. This can result in the inability to reach orgasm.

If you have your diabetes under control, you decrease your likelihood of these and many other problems that result from diabetes. You will also be able to manage many of these conditions by being able to make sure that you are controlling it. Natural methods can work just as well as prescription or over the counter drugs for your diabetes or the resulting afflictions themselves.

Taking the First Step:

Taking the first step into controlling your diabetes is recognizing that you have a problem and kindling the desire to make the needed lifestyle changes to fix it. start by changing what you eat, which will be the most effective method, and this book gives many wonderful recipes that can be used to naturally change what you're ingesting so that you can start to handle and control your diabetes. From smoothies to dinner recipes, there's always something that you can have that will help out while still delighting your taste buds.

Just remember that even though many diabetic recipes and remedies are great at helping with type one and two diabetes, most will help the best with just type two. Some won't even effect type one because of the severity of type on diabetes. However, a healthy lifestyle such as with your diet and exercise will always help, but talk to your doctor before adding any other remedies into your daily routine.

Chapter 2. Smoothie Recipes to Help Out

Everyone loves a good smoothie, and if you're diabetic, it doesn't mean that you have to cut them out. Of course, remember to handle everything with moderation, and smoothies can also be a meal replacement if they have enough nutrients and fiber or protein to help make sure that you stay full until your next meal. They're best for type two diabetes, and you'll find that many of them will help to make sure that you have the needed energy to exercise and control your weight, which is made both difficult and even more important when living with diabetes.

Smoothies are always fun, and many of these smoothies are aimed at type two diabetes. They range from green smoothies to tropical smoothies, so there is something to fit your taste buds. They're often used as a light snack by cutting down the serving size, and most recipes are aimed at making two to three smoothies, but not usually just one. It's always easier to stay on a diet, including the diabetic diet, if you have help.

Smoothie #1 The Green Light

Green smoothies are great for type two diabetes if you are careful with your ingredients and how much of your ingredients that you're using. When you are eating more raw fruits and vegetables then you're likely to cut your blood sugar levels in half over time. This smoothie can be made thicker with ice, but it's naturally sweet if you're using sweet berries.

Ingredients:

1. 2 Cups Baby Spinach, Shredded
2. ¼ Cup Chia Seeds, Soaked

3. 1 ½ Tablespoons Walnuts, Chopped
4. 1 Tablespoon Ground Flaxseed
5. 1 ½ Teaspoons Cinnamon, Ground
6. ½ Cup Blueberries, Fresh
7. 1 Scoop Vanilla Protein Powder, Sugar Free
8. ½ Cup Strawberries, Fresh or Frozen

Directions:

1. Put everything into your blender, and add water to blend until smooth. You can add ice as needed to make it thicker and make sure that everything is blended to the consistency that you're looking for.

Smoothie #2 Simple & Green

Sometimes, you don't always have the time to make a smoothie that requires a lot of ingredients. This is a great green smoothie to try for breakfast in the morning, and it only takes a few moments to make. Add a little Stevia or sugar free liquid sweetener to make sure it's sweet enough to start off your day with. Make sure your banana is ripe but not bruised for the best taste.

Ingredients:

1. 1 ½ Cups Water, Chilled
2. ½ Cup Ice
3. 1 Teaspoon Sweetener, Sugar Free
4. 1 Large Banana, Sliced & Frozen
5. 1/8 Ounce Hemp Seeds
6. ¼ Ounces Kale, Shredded
7. ¼ Ounces Baby Spinach, Shredded

Directions:

1. Just throw it all into the blender, and continue to blend until it's smooth, cold and ready to drink.

Smoothie #3 Savory & Satisfactory Green

This is yet another wonderful and simple diabetic smoothie recipe, which is best for type two diabetes. It's simple to make, and you can use it twice a day so long as you have a diabetic, traditional meal in-between.

Ingredients:

1. 1 Medium to Large Banana, Frozen & Sliced

2. ½ Small Avocado, Peeled & Cubed
3. 2 ½ Cups Baby Spinach, Shredded
4. ½ Cup Kale, Shredded
5. 1 Cup Almond Milk, Unsweetened & Chilled

Directions:

1. Throw it into the blender and make sure to blend away. Add a small amount of ice if you want your smoothie to be thicker.

Smoothie #4 Cheerful Cherry

You don't always want to have a green smoothie, and you don't need one just because you're diabetic. You can actually have a cheerful red cherry smoothie if you know the ingredients to put in, and this recipe does just the trick.

Ingredients:

1. 1 Cup Vanilla Almond Milk, Unsweetened & Chilled
2. ¾ Cup Greek Yogurt, Non-Fat & Blueberry

3. ½ Cup Blueberries, Fresh or Frozen
4. 1 ½ Cups Sweet Cherries, Pitted & Frozen
5. 1 Small Banana, Sliced & Frozen

Directions:

1. Blend until completely smooth, adding all ingredients together at the start. Remember that this is a smoothie recipe that makes four servings, so you can always put it in the freezer until later and blend again.

Smoothie #5 The Berry Blaster

Berries are delicious, and they're a great sweet treat, even if you're diabetic. This smoothie recipe is just like any other, and it has enough fruit to satisfy that sweet craving that you may be having.

Ingredients:

1. 2 Cups Strawberries, Frozen & Unsweetened
2. 1 Cup Blackberries, Fresh or Frozen
3. 1 Cup Raspberries, Fresh
4. 1 Cup Baby Spinach, Shredded
5. 1 Cup Pomegranate Juice, Chilled
6. 3 Tablespoons Vanilla Protein Powder, Sugar Free
7. 1 Tablespoon Honey, Raw

Directions:

1. Everything in this smoothie can be added together in your blender, and then you can cover and blend until smooth. You can add one more tablespoon honey if desired to sweeten a little more.

Smoothie #6 Plump Plum Smoothie

Plums aren't usually good out of season, but if you get the chance to get one in season when it's ripe, it's always great to add to the smoothie to get the sweet smoothie that you're looking for, especially when paired with banana and avocado, which is great if you're diabetic.

Ingredients:

1. ¼ Large Avocado, Peeled & Cubed
2. 1 Medium Banana, Sliced & Frozen
3. 1 Red Plum, Pitted & Peeled
4. 1 Cup Kale, Shredded
5. 1 Small Head Bok Choy, Chopped
6. 1 Teaspoon Honey, Raw

Direction:

Only add the teaspoon of honey if desired, but you can blend everything in this smoothie together.

Smoothie #7 Sweet Carrot Delight

You may not always think of carrots as sweet or diabetic friendly, but they are, especially when they're added into this recipe. From mango to carrots, this is a tropical smoothie recipe that shouldn't negatively impact your blood sugar levels, which will help you to control type two diabetes. If you want a colder, thicker smoothie than its best that you make your green tea in advance.

Ingredients:

1. 3 Cups Water
2. 1 Cup Baby Carrots, Peeled & Chopped
3. 1 Inch Ginger, Sliced Thin & Peeled
4. 4 Green Tea Bags
5. 1 ½ Teaspoons Honey, Raw
6. 1 Tablespoon Hemp Seeds
7. 2 Cups Mango, Chunked & Frozen

Directions:

1. Bring your water to a boil, and then insert the tea bags. Turn it to simmer, and let it simmer for three to six minutes.

2. Take out the teabags, and add the water and all other ingredients to the blender after the water has cooled. Blend until smooth.

Smoothie #8 Strawberry Banana Classic

Everyone loves the basic and classic strawberry banana smoothie, and you'll find that this is a diabetic friendly version that will still leave your mouth watering for more. You can use it once a day, but keep an eye on your blood sugar levels, as everyone is affected differently depending on how severe your diabetes is.

Ingredients:

1. 4 Cups Strawberries, Sliced & Chilled
2. ¾ Cup Low Fat Greek Yogurt, Vanilla
3. 1 Cup Ice Cubes
4. 1 Kiwi, Peeled & Sliced
5. 1 Medium Banana, Sliced & Frozen

Directions:

1. The kiwi is optional, but you can throw all ingredients into the blender. Just blend until it's smooth. Add less ice if you want it to be less thick.

Chapter 3. Herbal Remedies for Quick Control

One of the best ways to treat diabetes naturally is to try natural remedies, which are a great way to get your diabetes under control quickly. They will help on a day to day basis, but when you use herbal remedies on a regular basis, you will be able to control your diabetes in a more regular fashion. There are many herbal remedy options, and everyone has a preference towards different ones. Find a few that work for you, and work them into your daily routine.

Remedy #1 Cinnamon

This is a great natural remedy for diabetes because most people already have it in their spice cabinet, and if you don't, it's still quite easy to get ahold of. Cinnamon is known to help diabetes, and it can be critical to just use a half a teaspoon of cinnamon a day. It can be ground cinnamon, and you don't even need to take it on its own. It can mimic insulin, which will help to lower your need for insulin almost immediately. It's usually best to take cinnamon every morning if you want to help keep your diabetes under control. It can often your cell membranes, and ground cinnamon is easy to find.

Ingredients:

1. ½ Teaspoon Cinnamon
2. ½ Teaspoon Honey
3. 4 Ounces Water

Directions:

1. It may be best if you warm up the water, and then you can mix the cinnamon and honey together. Of course, you can also use cinnamon by adding it into your morning meal or even a morning drink or smoothie. Once mixed together, just drink once daily.

Remedy #2 Olive Oil

Olive oil is also something that you probably have in your kitchen, and you'll be able to find it in any grocery store if you need to get some. Make sure to get extra virgin olive oil if you want the best results in controlling your diabetes. Olive oil helps to reduce your blood levels, which will help you to control your diabetes as a benefit through the consumption of it.

You can even use it to prevent diabetes if consumed on a regular basis, and it can even help to prevent cardiovascular diseases. Monounsaturated fats, which olive oil consists of, is better for diabetes than saturated fats, which the majority of other oils consists of. It sadly does have 2,000 calories for every quarter cup, and you'll need to add that in to your daily calorie intake. Of course, you can cook with it a well, but it will not help as much as this direct herbal remedy.

Ingredients:

1. ¼ Cup Extra Virgin Olive Oil
2. ½ Teaspoon Cinnamon

Directions:

1. Just mix it all together, and drink it once in the evening before bed.

Remedy #3 Billberry

Billberry is actually a relative to the blueberry, and it has many antioxidants in both the leaves and the fruit. They help to prevent the damage to your small blood Vessels, which can damage your eye's retinas and cause nerve pain. Bilberry will help to lower blood sugar when taken properly, and it can help to prevent this damage which you're at an increased risk of with diabetes.

Ingredients:

1. 80 Milligrams Bilberry Extract

Directions:

1. Take daily. It can be 80 to 120 milligrams two times per day. You need to have a standardized bilberry extract for this to work. Many people will get this in supplement form to make it easier, but it can sometimes be harder to find.

Remedy #4 Ginseng

A ginseng tincture usually works best, but you'll find that a capsule will work as well. Green tea with ginseng has been known to help work in lowering your blood sugar and controlling diabetes as well. This is because ginseng slows carbohydrate absorption. Which will increase your cell's ability to actually use glucose, and this can increase insulin secretion from your pancreas. It also has the added effect of boosting your immune system. You can lower your blood glucose using a simple ginseng capsule.

Ingredients:

1. 3 to 5 Millimeters Tincture

Directions:

1. If you're using the tincture, takes it three times daily to lower your blood glucose about fifteen to twenty percent. Of course, you can take one to three grams a day in a tablet form if you prefer, which many people find is a little easier when dealing with ginseng for diabetes.

Remedy #5 Prickly Pear Cactus

This is actually a fruit you can eat to help you control your diabetes, but you can also find it in a capsule form to make it a little easier if you prefer. Many people can find a prickly pear cactus at their local farmer's market or at your grocery store. If you can't, then just run over to a natural food or health store to make sure that you get the capsule you need to make sure you have your diabetes under control quickly and effectively.

It will help to lower your blood sugar, and the ripe fruit is usually best. You can even use the juice or powder if it's easier to find. If so, then just follow the directions on the label. It has a component that helps to work similarly as insulin, which will help lower your blood sugar, but the fruit also contains a lot of fiber, making it the perfect diabetic snack as well.

Ingredients:

1. ½ Cup Prickly Pear Cactus

Directions:

1. Aim to eat a half cup a day, and you can split it up and use it as one or two snacks, or even incorporate it into your breakfast or lunch. However, make sure that it's cooked. Many people will cook it at 350 until softened with a little bit of lemon or lime juice sprinkled over it.

Remedy #6 Bitter Melon

Bitter melon is yet another wonderful thing to add to your daily routine if you want to control your diabetes. You need to find the juice to do so, and so it's usually best to run to a health food store if you don't want to buy it online. Make sure that you're getting a quality product, and that no sugar has been added for it to actually help you. It can help to lower your blood sugar by blocking sugar absorption in your intestines. Just remember that using this herbal remedy can cause a side effect of gastrointestinal problems. If you are experiencing gastrointestinal problems, talk to your doctor immediately and stop taking bitter melon.

Ingredients:

1. 4 Tablespoon Bitter Melon Juice

Directions:

1. You can take three to six tablespoons of bitter melon juice every day to help with your diabetes, but most people stick to four. Otherwise, you can use a capsule form and follow the instructions on the bottle.

Chapter 4. Dinner Recipes That Will Work

Dinner is an important meal of the day to almost everyone, so it's important that you have a diabetic friendly dinner that doesn't disappoint your taste buds. If you are unhappy with what you are eating, you're more likely to eat foods that are going to hurt you because of your diabetes rather than help you. That's why it's important that you find the right recipes for you that still make sure that you're controlling your diabetes in a natural way, and the recipes below should help.

Recipe #1 Roasted Salmon

Salmon is a great diabetic food, and fish is always healthy for your body, especially your brain and heart. Of course, with the right ingredients, it makes a complete diabetic meal that you can make even when people are coming over. It's sure to delight any who love the fresh taste that salmon has to offer.

Ingredients:

1. ¼ Cup Heavy Whipping Cream
2. 2 Tablespoons White Wine Vinegar
3. 2 Tablespoons Dill Fresh & Chopped
4. 1 ½ Teaspoons Buttermilk
5. 1 1/8 Teaspoons Sea Salt, Divided
6. 1 1/8 Teaspoons Black Pepper, Ground & Divided
7. 2 Tablespoons Shallots, Chopped Fine
8. 2 Tablespoons Parsley, chopped
9. 3 Tablespoons Olive Oil
10. 3 Pounds Salmon Fillet
11. 3 Tablespoons Capers, Chopped & Drained
12. ¼ Horseradish, Grated Fine

Directions:

1. The buttermilk, ream, and vinegar should be combined in a small bowl, and then you'll want to cover it, usually with plastic wrap. Let it sit at room temperature for eight hours before stirring in the dill, an eight a teaspoon of salt and pepper. Refrigerate, keeping it there overnight.
2. Combine the salt, pepper, horseradish, shallow, olive oil, capers, and parsley together in a small bowl. Spread this mixture over your salmon, making sure it's even. Also refrigerate overnight.
3. The oven will need to be turned to 450.
4. The skin side of your fish should be placed down on a prepared pan. It should be on a baking sheet that is lined with parchment paper, and should be

baked for thirteen minutes before being removed from the oven.
5. The broiler should then be preheated to high, and then you can broil the fish for five minutes. Cut it into eight portions, and serve with the dill sauce.

Recipe #2 Taco Pizza Fiesta

If you're looking for something a little more casual, taco pizza, especially this deep dish recipe, is great. It is also wonderful for parties, and it may be diabetic friendly but it packs a punch to your taste buds that you aren't going to forget anytime soon.

Ingredients:

1. 1 lb Ground Beef
2. 15 Ounces Canned Tomatoes with Green chilies, Diced & Drained
3. 10 Ounces Refrigerated Pizza Dough
4. 4 Ounces Mozzarella Cheese, Part-Skim & Shredded
5. 1/8 Cup Salsa
6. 1/8 Cup Sour Cream Reduced Fat
7. 1 Teaspoon Mexican Seasoning, Salt Free
8. ½ Cup Chopped Onion, Frozen

Directions:

1. The oven needs preheated to 425.
2. The beef and onion will need to be cooked over medium-high heat together until your beef is browned. You need to stir to crumble while cooking, and then drain it well. Return it all to the pan, and add in your seasoning as well as your tomatoes, cooking over medium-high heat one again for at least one minute or until it's heated all the way through. Then, set it aside.
3. The pizza crust will need to b unrolled, and put in a thirteen by nine inch baking dish that's been coated with cooking spray. It should be pressed to the bottom and come halfway up the sides. Spoon in your beef mixture.
4. Bake for twelve minutes in the oven, and then top it with your cheese, baking for another five. The cheese should melt and

the edges of the crust should be browned already. Let it stand five minutes.
5. Slice to serve once it's cooled for about five minutes, topping with sour cream and salsa for those who want it.

Recipe #3 Turkey Stir Fry

Turkey or chicken are both great, but turkey gives you a unique flavor to this broccoli stir fry. Turkey tenderloins are best, but you can use turkey cutlets. Turkey breast will work as well in a pinch.

Ingredients:

1. 2 Teaspoons Sesame Oil, Divided
2. 1 Cup Low Sodium Chicken Broth, Fat Free
3. 5 Garlic Cloves, Minced
4. 1 lb Turkey Tenderloins, Cut into Strips
5. 1 ½ Tablespoons Cornstarch
6. ¼ Teaspoon Sea Salt, Fine
7. ¼ Teaspoon Crushed Red Pepper
8. 1 Red Bell Pepper, Cut into Strips
9. 2 Cups Broccoli Florets
10. 8 Ounces Canned Water Chestnuts, Drained & Sliced
11. 2 Tablespoons Soy Sauce, Low Sodium

Directions:

1. Take a skillet, placing it over medium-high heat, and add a teaspoon of sesame oil into the pan. Make sure the pan is coated evenly before you add the turkey and fry up for five minutes. There should be no pink in the middle whenyou're done, and then you can remove it to cool and set it to the side.
2. The broth, garlic, cornstarch, and red pepper, and salt should then be added together. Make sure the all of the cornstarch dissolves before setting it aside.
3. Take another teaspoon of oil, putting it into the pan, and put in the broccoli and

red pepper. Fry up for one minute, and add the water chestnuts, frying for another thirty seconds to a minute, turning it to high heat.
4. Add in the broth mixture, and put it with the turkey, juices, and soy sauce. Bring it to a boil for one to two minutes until its thickened, stirring in vegetables as well.

Recipe #4 Steak & Fried Rice

If you love steak, you don't have to give it up just because you're diabetic. When paired with fried rice it's simply delightful, and you'll find that this amazing recipe is taste friendly as well as being diabetic friendly.

Ingredients:

1. 2 Eggs, Beaten Lightly
2. 2 Tablespoons Ginger, Fresh Grated
3. 4 Garlic Cloves, Minced
4. 1 Cup Peas, Frozen
5. 12 Ounces Broccoli Coleslaw Mix
6. 2 Cups Brown Rice, Cooked
7. 4 Green Onions Sliced Small
8. 4 Tablespoons Soy Sauce, Low Sodium & Divided
9. ¾ lb Sirloin Steak, Cut into Thin Strips
10. 2 Teaspoons Olive oil

Directions:

1. Put a large pan over medium heat, cooking the eggs after coating it with a cooking spray or a little more olive oil. Break up the eggs by scrambling it into small pieces, and remove them from the pan. Set aside until needed later.
2. Heat the oil, making sure the pan is over medium-high heat, and then add in your beef. Stir fry until no longer pink. It should take one to two minutes.
3. Then, add in your soy sauce, mixing it together before removing both from the pan.
4. Take the coleslaw mix, garlic, ginger, and peas, cooking together until crisp

and tender. Add in your cooked rice, remaining soy sauce, and toss it all to combine. Keep it over heat until it is all heated, stirring in the eggs, green onions, and beef.
5. Serve while warm.

Recipe #5 One Dish Pork Chops

When cooked right, you don't even have to give up pork chops if you're diabetic. You'll find that this is a lovely recipe, and what's even better about it is that it's one dish, making it that much easier to make.

Ingredients:

1. 1/3 Cup All Purpose Flour, Divided
2. ¼ Teaspoon Sea Salt, Fine
3. 1/8 Teaspoon Black Pepper, Ground
4. 8 Boneless Pork Loin Chops, ½ Inch Thick
5. ¼ Cup Butter, Cubed
6. 2 lbs Small Red Potatoes
7. 1 lb Whole Onions, Canned & Drained
8. 1 lb Carrots, Cut in 2-3 Inch Pieces & Peeled
9. 7 Cups Cabbage, Shredded
10. 2 Cups Apple Juice

Directions:

1. Take a ¼ cup of the flour, pepper, salt and pork chops, putting it in a zip locked bag and closing it. Shake until the pork chops are coated, and then put your pork chops in a Dutch oven, with medium-high heat, browning your pork chops on both sides. Set aside, and keep them warm.
2. Take the remaining flour and your pan drippings, blending them together in a bowl, and then whisk in your apple juice. Bring the mixture to a boil, and stir it while cooking for two minutes. It should thicken.

3. Return the pork chops to the pan, adding onions, carrots, and potatoes. Cover, and bake at 350 for a half hour.
4. Top it with cabbage, covering it and putting it back into the oven for fifty minutes to one hour. The vegetables should be tender, baste with the apple juice mixture throughout.

Recipe #6 Spiced Salmon

Once again, salmon is great, and it's even better for your health, even as a diabetic. That's why you'll find that salmon recipes are commonly used, and it's a fish that takes to flavor rather easily.

Ingredients:

1. ½ Teaspoon Ginger, Ground
2. ½ Teaspoon Garam Masaia
3. ¾ Teaspoon Coriander, Ground
4. ¼ Teaspoon Se Salt, Fine
5. 1/8 Teaspoon Ground Red Pepper
6. 4 Skinless Salmon Fillets, Six Ounces
7. ¼ Teaspoon Turmeric, Ground

Directions:

1. Make sure to preheat your broiler, and then combine your ginger, coriander, turmeric, salt, pepper, garam masala, and your ground red pepper together. Rube the spice mixture over your salmon.
2. Take a baking sheet, coating it with cooking spray, and spread your salmon over it. Cover it with foil, broiling for seven minutes.
3. Remove the foil, and broil for another four.

Recipe #7 Ginger Vegetables & Grilled Shrimp

With moderation, you can even have shrimp, especially with these healthy ginger vegetables that are sure to make an impact on your taste buds. This is a dish that is good for those simple nights or even if you have friends over. It has an exotic, and yet deeply satisfying taste.

Ingredients:

1. 1 Cup Mushrooms, Sliced
2. ½ Cup Red Bell Pepper, Sliced
3. 4 Cloves Garlic, Minced
4. ½ Cup Green Bell Peppers, Sliced
5. 2 Cups Broccoli Florets

6. 1 Cup Cooked Brown Rice
7. 1 Tablespoon Olive Oil, Divided
8. 3 Teaspoons Brown Sugar
9. 1 Tablespoons Cornstarch
10. 1 Tablespoon Water
11. 1 Tablespoon Seasoned Rice Vinegar
12. 1 ½ lbs Shrimp, Raw & Cleaned
13. 5 Green Onions, Sliced
14. 3 Tablespoons Soy Sauce, Low Sodium
15. 1 Tablespoon Fresh ginger, Grated

Directions:

1. Take a medium bowl, combine your water, brown sugar, cornstarch, rice vinegar, ginger, and soy sauce.

2. Spray a large skillet with cooking spray, putting it over medium high heat, and then add in about two teaspoons of oil. When it's hot, add in your shrimp and sauté for about four to six minutes. It should be fully cooked, and then you can remove it from the skillet, setting it aside for later.
3. Take a teaspoon of oil and your garlic, sautéing it for one minute before adding in peppers, broccoli, mushrooms and green onions. Fry for five to eight minutes. The vegetables should become tender.
4. Add your soy sauce mixture, and cook. Stir constantly until it all thickens.
5. Add the shrimp back in, cooking until heated, and serve over cooked rice while warm.

Chapter 5. Snacks & A Few Extra Recipes

Snacks and a few extra recipes are always welcome when you're learning how to eat healthy while being a diabetic. You'll find that it helps to make sure that you have everything you need to feel comfortable on a natural, healthy diet that will help to make sure that you feel you aren't missing out on anything. These dessert and snack recipes are sure to help.

Recipe #1 Tiramisu

This is a light version of tiramisu, and it's perfectly healthy. It's great to add to any diet, diabetic or not. This popular Italian dessert is still as moist as it is creamy, allowing it to delight your senses.

Ingredients:

1. ¼ cup Water

2. ½ Cup Boiling Water
3. 1 Tablespoon Instant Coffee Granules
4. ½ Teaspoon Baking Cocoa
5. 2 Packages Ladyfingers, Split & 3 Ounces Each
6. 3 Large Egg Whites
7. ½ Cup White Sugar
8. 1 Tablespoon White Sugar
9. 1 ½ Cups Whipped Topping, Reduced & Divided
10. 2/3 Cup Confectioner's Sugar, Divided
11. 8 Ounces Cream Cheese, Reduced Fat
12. 2 Tablespoons Coffee Liqueur

Directions:

1. Take a small bowl, beating your confectioners' sugar and cream cheese together until it becomes smooth. Fold in a cup of the whipped topping before setting it aside.
2. Take a half a cup of the white sugar, the egg whites, and the water, putting them in a small saucepan. The heat should be turned to low. Beat at a low speed for a minute, and continue to beat over low heat. The temperature should reach 160, so you'll be beating for eight to ten minutes before pulling it into a large bowl. Beat it on high, and stiff peaks should form. It'll take about six to eight minutes. Fold it into your cream cheese mixture.
3. Arrange half of your ladyfingers into an eleven by seven inch dish that's ungreased. Combine the coffee liqueur,

coffee granules, and all remaining sugar together. Brush it over your lady fingers. Top with the cream cheese mixture, but only half of it. Repeat, and then sprinkle with cocoa.
4. Refrigerate for at least two hours before serving.

Recipe #2 Strawberry Parfait

This diabetic recipe can be great for a dessert, breakfast, or even as just a snack. It's healthy, and it provides you the needed nutrients, such as calcium and vitamin D. there's no reason to limit your flavor just because of diabetes. You can choose any other yogurt flavor as well to spice up this parfait just a little bit more. Just try to make sure it's Greek Yogurt without too much sugar.

Ingredients:

1. 6 Ounces Low Fat Greek Yogurt, Strawberry
2. ½ Cup Strawberries, Sliced
3. ¼ Cup Granola, Without Raisins

Directions:

1. Take a large glass jar or mug, and layer all of the ingredients. Start with the fruit on the bottom, some of the yogurt, more fruit, more yogurt, and top with the granola. Dig in when you're ready, but keep it chilled until then.

Recipe #3 Almond Butter

Almond butter is a great way to make sure that you have everything you need for a quick and easy snack. It's much better for you than peanut butter, but you can use hazelnut butter and walnut butter as well. Many people will use fruit to dip the almond butter into, and that's a great snack or even a great breakfast. Almond butter can help to control blood sugar spikes, and it'll help you to control your diabetes.

Ingredients:

1. 3 Cups Almonds
2. 2 Teaspoons Honey, Raw

Directions:

1. Blend on high in a food processor. It's best to use an S blade, and you'll need to scrape the sides periodically. Blend for twenty-five to thirty-five minutes.
2. Add in honey, and blend for another three to five minutes. It should be smooth and creamy. Store it in an airtight glass jar until you're ready to use it.

Recipe #4 Diabetic Trail Mix

One again, almonds play a key role in this trail mix, and you even have some cinnamon in there to help you with your blood sugar levels as well. A half cup serving is usually best.

Ingredients:

1. 2 Teaspoons Cinnamon, Ground
2. 4 Cups Vegetable Sticks, Mixed & Crisp

3. 2 Cups Corn Square Cereal
4. 2 Cups Toasted Oat Cereal
5. 1 ¾ Cups Pretzels, Bite Size
6. ½ Teaspoon Chili Powder
7. ½ Cup Almonds, Whole
8. 1 Teaspoon Brown Sugar, Packed
9. 1 Teaspoon Paprika, Ground
10. ½ Teaspoon Cumin, Ground
11. ¼ Teaspoon Cayenne Pepper
12. ¼ Teaspoon Sea Salt, Fine

Directions:

1. Preheat your oven. It should be at 300 degrees. Take a roasting pan, and put in

your cereals, almonds, pretzels, and vegetable sticks.
2. In a bowl, combine your paprika, chili powder, cumin, cayenne pepper, salt, and brown sugar together. Coat your other mixture in it, and then toss it with cooking spray. Make sure it's all coated well, and place in the roasting pan.
3. Bake for eighteen to twenty minutes. You should stir twice, and then spread it out to cool. Store in an airtight container, and it should last up to a week.

Recipe #5 Roasted Nuts

Roasted nuts are great for diabetes. They're great at making sure your blood sugar doesn't spike, and this roasted nut recipe is no different. It even tastes great due to the wonderful seasoning that also helps to make sure that your blood sugar is under control. Try using a brown sugar substitute to make it even biter if your diabetes is a little more severe.

Ingredients:

1. 1 Egg White
2. 1 Tablespoon Water
3. 1/8 Teaspoon Cayenne Pepper

4. 1 Teaspoon Garlic Salt
5. 1 Cup Whole Cashews, Raw
6. 1 Cup Whole Almonds, Raw
7. 1 Cup Whole Walnuts, Halved & Raw
8. 1 Cup Pecan Halves, Raw
9. 3 Tablespoons Brown Sugar Substitute, Packed
10. 1 Tablespoon Cumin, Ground
11. 2 Tablespoons Chili Powder

Directions:

1. The oven needs to be set to 300, and then you'll want to take out a medium bowl. Combine your water and egg white

together, and beat it until frothy with a fork.
2. Coat your nuts in the mixture, and let it stand for five to six minutes.
3. Take a large plastic bag that's sealable, and combine your brown sugar substitute, garlic salt, cumin, chili powder, and cayenne pepper. Add in your nuts, shaking to coat.
4. Take a 15x10x1 inch baking pan, and spread your nuts in it evenly. Place it in the oven baking for thirty-five to forty minutes. The nuts should be completely dry when they're done. Stir twice in between.
5. Spread them out to dry, and a quarter cup is a serving size. Remember to keep at room temperature in an airtight container.

Recipe #6 Trail Mix Balls

Sometimes, you don't just want to munch on random nuts. So you'll find that these trail mix balls are just fine. It even will help with your diabetes, and it'll keep your blood sugar from spiking.

Ingredients:

1. ½ Teaspoon Vanilla Extract
2. ¾ Cup Rolled Oats, Toasted
3. 1/3 Cup Dried Fruit
4. ¼ Cup Peanuts, Lightly Salted
5. ¼ Cup Large Flake Coconut, Unsweetened

6. 1 Tablespoon Sesame Seeds
7. ¼ Cup Sunflower Seed Kernels
8. 1/3 Cup Almond Butter
9. 2 Tablespoons Water
10. 1/3 Cup Honey, Raw
11. ¾ Cup Rice Cereal, Crisp

Directions:

1. Take a small saucepan, putting the water and honey together over low heat. Stir to combine, and then remove from heat.
2. Add in your almond butter and vanilla, whisk it until the almond butter is melted and it's all smooth.

3. Take a large bowl, adding your oats, fruit bits, peanuts, sunflower seed kernels, rice cereal, coconut, and sesame seeds. Pour the honey mixture over it, and coat it by stirring. Let chill for one or two hours. It should be firm.
4. Take damp hands, and shape it into thirty small balls. Chill the balls, and store in an airtight container in the refrigerator.

Chapter 6. Herbal Teas That Produce Results

Herbal teas are also a great way to make sure that you have your diabetes under control. Tea is known to help prove your insulin sensitivity, so it's a great thing to add to your daily diet if you're a diabetic. It will also help with a healthy blood pressure and it can help you reduce your risk of developing diabetes in the first place. You'll want black tea, green tea, or even oolong to enjoy these benefits. Just remember never to add milk, as it'll reduce the effects that it has on your insulin sensitivity.

Raw honey is also good. As a diabetic, you shouldn't eat sugars, but honey, when raw, is a little different. It's not the same as other sweeteners, and it can actually help you to control both your sweet tooth and your blood sugar levels. Of course, raw honey is different than just any honey you might pick up at the grocery store. Many honeys are actually infused with sugar, so instead go for raw or organic. Local honey is usually raw honey, and you can get it at the local farmer's market.

Tea #1 Cinnamon Green Tea

Cinnamon and green tea is going to help you to lower your blood sugar, and this is a great green tea recipe. It'll help to make sure you keep your diabetes under control.

Ingredients:

1. 2 Tablespoons Green Tea Leaves
2. 1 Teaspoon Cinnamon, Ground
3. 1 Teaspoon Honey, Raw

Directions:

1. Boil a cup of water, and then place in your green tea leaves and cinnamon. Bring it down to a simmer, and let simmer for five to six minutes.
2. Strain the mixture, and then add in honey while still warm. Drink warm.

Tea #2 Rosemary Green Tea

Rosemary is known to help fight diabetes, and using fresh herbs is always best. Of course, if you aren't growing rosemary yourself, they can be hard to get ahold of, so you'll find that dried rosemary will do fine in a pinch. Add a little bit of cinnamon for added flavor, and drink at least once daily.

Ingredients:

1. 2 Tablespoon Green Tea Leaves
2. ½ Tablespoon Cinnamon, Ground
3. 1 Teaspoon Honey, Raw
4. 2 Teaspoons Rosemary, Dried

Directions:

1. Boil one cup of water, and then put in all of your herbs, including your cinnamon as you reduce it to a simmer for six to seven minutes.
2. Strain out the herbs, and add in your honey. Mix until the honey is completely dissolved, and drink while warm.

Tea #3 Lemongrass Tea Mix

Lemongrass is actually known for helping with diabetes as well since it'll help to control your blood sugar. It's even known to lower your cholesterol and help to prevent heart disease. Of course, with a little peppermint, and just a dash of honey, this is a great tea to try.

Ingredients:

1. 1 Oolong Tea Bag
2. 2 Tablespoons Lemongrass, Dried
3. 3-4 Mint Leaves, Fresh (Or ½ Teaspoon Peppermint Extract)
4. ½ Teaspoon Honey, Raw

Directions:

1. Boil a cup of water, adding in your tea bag, mint leaves, and lemongrass too steep as you reduce it to a simmer. Let

simmer for four to six minutes, and then strain.
2. Add in honey, and serve while warm.

Tea #4 Spiced Black Tea

As stated before, you'll find that black tea is great at controlling your blood sugar. With honey and cinnamon, you're sure to get a rich, spiced tea that will help to make sure that you control your blood sugar. Of course, cloves are known to help with diabetes as well.

Ingredients:

1. 2 Tablespoons Black Tea Leaves
2. 1 Teaspoon Cinnamon, Ground
3. 1 Teaspoon Honey, Raw
4. ½ Teaspoon Ginger, Ground
5. ½ Teaspoon Cloves, Ground

Ingredients:

1. Boil one cup of water, and add in all of your ingredients except your honey.

Reduce it to a simmer, and simmer for about six to seven minutes.
2. Strain, and then add in the honey. Make sure to stir until it's dissolved, and then you can serve warm.

Tea #5 Oolong Delight

Oolong and black tea are good for you, add in cinnamon, cloves, and honey and this is a great evening tea mixture. It's not as light and airy tasting as what you'd want for during the day, but you'll find it's great when you're relaxing in the evening. Add less cloves if desired, but remember that cloves help your blood sugar levels, so find the right mix for you.

Ingredients:

1. 1 Tablespoon Black Tea Leaves
2. 1 Tablespoon Oolong Tea Leaves
3. 2 Teaspoons Cloves, Ground
4. ½ Teaspoon Cinnamon
5. 1 Teaspoon Honey, Raw
6. ½ Teaspoon Lemon Juice, Fresh

Directions:

1. Boil one cup of water, and then add in all ingredients except your lemon juice and honey.
2. Turn down to let it simmer for five to seven minutes, and then strain.
3. While warm, add in honey and lemon juice. Stir to combine and then serve warm.

Tea #6 Refreshing Green Tea

If you're looking for a morning tea, then you're most likely looking for a green tea. This wonderful green tea is refreshing with its crisp taste of rosemary and mint, which is known to help keep your blood sugar levels in check.

Ingredients:

1. 2 Tablespoons Green Tea Leaves
2. 1 Tablespoon Rosemary, Dried
3. 4-6 Mint Leaves, Fresh
4. ½ Teaspoon Honey, Raw

Directions:

1. Boil a cup of water, and then add rosemary, mint leaves, and green tea.
2. Reduce to a simmer, and let simmer for five to six minutes.
3. Take off heat, and strain.
4. Add in honey, stirring until dissolved. Serve warm or let cool and serve over ice.

Tea #7 Sage & Rosemary Tea

Sage is also known to help with diabetes by keeping your blood sugar levels under control. It can even help to boost your immune system and keep headaches at bay. When paired with rosemary, you have an earthy tea that is sure to delight your taste buds.

Ingredients:

1. 1 ½ Tablespoons Rosemary, Dried
2. 2 Tablespoons Sage, Dried
3. 1 Teaspoon Honey, Raw

Directions:

1. Boil a single cup of water, and then add your rosemary and sage. Reduce it from a boil to a simmer, allowing to simmer for four to six minutes. Take it off heat, and strain.
2. While warm, add honey and drink once dissolved.

Chapter 7. Herbal Supplements for Strong Results

You should always talk to your doctor before you add any new pill to your daily regime, especially if it can lower your blood sugar, which most of these supplements can do. If so, you'll need to check your blood sugar more often, and your medication dosages, if you are taking any at the time, may need to be altered.

You should see results in a month or two, but with herbal supplements when trying to control diabetes, you're going to need to wait until then. Immediate results will not be seen. Not every supplement will work for every person, so you'll find that you may need to do some trial and error. If you do not see results within a few months, then you may want to switch to a different want by reevaluating it with your doctor.

Supplement #1 Gymnema Sylvestre

This is a supplement that is great at lowering your blood sugar, and you'll usually take it twice daily with a dosage of 200 to 250 milligrams. It's known as a sugar destroyer, and it'll reduce your ability to detect sweetness. It's a blood sugar control that is meant to work quickly, and it helps your cells to use glucose, and it does this by stimulating your production of insulin. It doesn't have any known serious side effects, so it's a supplement that is relatively harmless to take.

Supplement #2 Magnesium

One of the best parts about taking magnesium to help control your blood sugar is that it's actually easy to get ahold of, so you won't have to search for it, and you usually don't have to worry about quality so long as you get it from a health store. It's also only taken once per day, so it's easy to work into your daily schedule. A typical dosage is anywhere from 250 to 350 milligrams, and many people that have diabetes actually has a magnesium deficiency. You can ask your doctor to test for this deficiency, and it can worsen high blood sugar as well as insulin resistance. Magnesium will help to lower your blood sugar levels while improving insulin function. Before adding it, make sure you have a magnesium deficiency, or it'll provide you with no results.

Supplement #3 Chromium

This is yet another supplement that is great at lowering your blood sugar, and it's yet another one that only needs to be taken once a day in 200 micrograms. It's a trace mineral, and it's supposed to help enhance the action taken by insulin. It is known to help you normalize blood sugar levels, but you have to be deficient in chromium. Otherwise, this is a supplement that will do nothing to help you. Many people who are suffering from diabetes are suffering from a chromium deficiency, but it's best to have your doctor test for it before taking it.

Supplement #4 Gamma-Linolenic Acid

This is known to ease the nerve pain that diabetes can cause, and if you aren't having nerve pain, then you shouldn't actually take it. Always talk to your doctor before taking it, and it should only be taken once daily. A typical dosage is 270 milligrams to 540, and you'll need to talk to your doctor about what's right for you. Taking this supplement can even prevent nerve pain associated with diabetes, so your doctor may suggest it if you're at risk.

Supplement #5 Fenugreek

This is yet another supplement that is great at lowering blood sugar, and it's usually taken with each meal. It can be five to thirty grams with that meal. The seeds are commonly found in Indian cooking, and it can increase insulin sensitivity. It is also known to help reduce high cholesterol as an added benefit. Fenugreek also has an amino acid in it that is known to boost the release of insulin. This can help you to improve your blood sugar. It can especially help you avoid post meal spikes in blood sugar levels.

Supplement #6 Alpha-Lipoic Acid

This isn't just a supplement for lowering blood sugar even though it can help with that. It can also ease the nerve pain associated with diabetes. A typical dosage is anywhere from 600 to 800 milligrams once daily, and it helps to neutralize free radicals. A free radical build up, which can be caused by having too high of blood sugar, can damage your nerves as well as cause other problems. It can help your cells to take up the blood sugar, decreasing the buildup of high blood sugar. This will also help to improve insulin sensitivity and relieve burning and numbness.

Supplement #7 Cinnamon

Sometimes, you may just not like the taste of cinnamon, but it doesn't stop cinnamon from being helpful in controlling your blood sugar levels and therefore controlling your diabetes. You'll find that taking a cinnamon supplement can help you, and it has no serious side effects, but for some people it does upset their stomach. It can help to improve your blood sugar level, but it should have no sugar in it. Just follow the directions on the bottle, and you'll find your blood sugar levels are a little more stable when it's taken once daily.

Supplement #8 Vanadium

Vanadium is also a trace mineral, and it can help with your blood sugar levels if you're a diabetic. It's actually known to mimic insulin, which will help you to keep your blood sugar levels under control without unusual spikes. A suggested dose of vanadium is 100 milligrams daily, but you need to talk to your doctor. It's also known as vanadyl sulfate.

Supplement #9 Berberine

Berberine can be a helpful supplement, and it's a plant alkaloid which targets AMP-activated protein kinase. It's a regulator of the metabolism, and it stimulates your cells to take in glucose and improve your insulin sensitivity. It can reduce glucose production in the liver, which is usually in overdrive with diabetic patients. A recommended dose is 1,600 milligrams daily, but only once a day. It's usually best to take in the mornings.

Supplement #10 Vitamin E

This may seem like a simple supplement, but it can help many people suffering from diabetes. It's relatively safe to take, but always remember to talk to your doctor before adding any supplement into your daily routine, as almost any supplement has the ability to interact with some medication. Vitamin E is a fat soluble antioxidant, and it can help to improve your glucose control while protecting blood vessels as well as nerves from free radical damage. Free radical damage is often accelerated by diabetes, and having high doses of vitamin E will help to reverse the effects. Of course, it's usually recommended that you take 300 IUs, but always talk to your doctor first.

Supplement #11 Banaba Leaf Extract

Banaba leaf extract comes from Asia, and it actually has colosolic acid. This can help to promote the transport of glucose into cells, which can keep your blood sugars levels even throughout the day. Usually you only need three milligrams of banaba leaf daily, and you should be able to get it from a local health food store.

Chapter 8. Some Bonus Recipes to Try

Diabetes is commonly controlled by what you're taking into your body, from teas to supplements to food, and that's why it's important to stay with a diet that is diabetic friendly. It's easier if you have a wealth of recipes at your disposal, which is why these bonus recipes are meant to help you stay on track with controlling your diabetes in a natural way.

Bonus Recipe #1 No Bake Chocolate Mint

This is a diabetic dessert recipe that has 24 servings in it, so you'll need to cut it into twenty-four pieces. One bar is a piece, and it has a minty and chocolatey flavor. You don't need to worry about baking it, so it's considered easy and fun to make.

Ingredients:

1. 1 Teaspoon Sea Salt, Fine
2. ¾ Cup Powdered Sugar
3. 2 Ounces Cream Cheese, Softened & Reduced Fat
4. ½ Teaspoon Peppermint Extract
5. ½ Teaspoon Shortening
6. 6 Tablespoons Butter, Unsalted
7. 1 Cup Rolled Oats, Quick Cooking
8. ½ Cup Dark Chocolate Pieces
9. 1 Cup Crushed Chocolate Wafers
10. 1 Tablespoon Milk, Fat Free
11. 1 Tablespoon Cocoa Powder, Unsweetened

Directions:

1. Get an eight by eight by two baking pan, preparing it by spraying it likely with cooking spray. Then, set it aside.
2. Take the oats and place them in a food processor, grinding them fine to place on the bottom as crust. First, you'll want to get a ¼ cup of the chocolate pieces, butter, and the oats, combining them in a saucepan over low heat and stirring until melted. Combine your wafers, cocoa powder, milk and your salt. This is your crust mixture, which you'll place into the bottom of the pan. Let it chill in the fridge for about fifteen minutes.
3. Take the same saucepan and take a ¼ cup of the chocolate pieces, and the shortening, placing them together. Heat until melted, and set it aside.
4. Take a medium bowl, placing in your peppermint extract, cream cheese and

powdered sugar. Blend until smooth, and put it over the crust.
5. Drizzle in your chocolate mixture, and chill for another hour. Sprinkle with fresh mint if desired.

Bonus Recipe #2 Applesauce Popsicles

If you're in the middle of hot weather, then you'll love this diabetic sweet treat that is good for any hot day. You'll need to prepare them in advance, but with a Popsicle tray they're easy to make, and they taste great. Just remember that each pop is a serving, and this recipe should make sixteen.

Ingredients:

1. 32 Ounces Applesauce, Unsweetened
2. 3 Tablespoons Honey, Raw
3. ½ Cup Strawberries, Sliced
4. ½ Cup Blackberries, Fresh
5. ½ Cup Blueberries, Fresh
6. ½ Cup Raspberries, Fresh

Directions:

1. Take a large bowl, combining all ingredients together, making sure the honey is swirled throughout.
2. Spoon the mixture into sixteen containers, and then cover to freeze overnight. You can use five ounce paper cups as well, but remember to cover in plastic wrap either way. Make sure to insert a Popsicle stick into each before freezing, and then you can just take them out to eat when you like.

Bonus Recipe #3 Baked Apple Slices

This is a great dessert that can be done in only a few minutes, and it's easy to make. You only need three ingredients, and have your oven ready at 350. Just choose an apple of your choice, but usually a yellow or red apple works best.

Ingredients:

1. 1 Small Apple
2. 1 ½ Teaspoons Honey, Raw
3. 1 Teaspoon Cinnamon, Ground

Directions:

1. Slice your apple, but do not peel it. Turn your oven to 350, and then lightly spray a baking sheet down with cooking spray.
2. Place your apple slices on it, and drizzle with honey, sprinkling with cinnamon.
3. Bake at 350 until soft, and let cool before serving.

Bonus Recipe #4 Diabetic Peanut Butter Cookies

Everyone loves peanut butter cookies, and you can have them so long as you only have one to two coolies. Try with one with this diabetic recipe until you find how it reacts and causes your blood sugar levels to react. Of course, it's just as sweet as any other peanut butter recipe.

Ingredients:

1. ¾ Cup Peanut Butter
2. ¼ Cup Almond Butter
3. 1 Cup Splenda
4. 2 Teaspoons Cinnamon, Ground
5. 1 Large Egg
6. 1 Teaspoon Vanilla

Directions:

1. Take a large bowl, beating all ingredients together until smooth.
2. Preheat your oven to 350, and prepare a baking sheet by spraying it down with cooking spray.
3. Roll the dough into balls, and then press down until flat.
4. Bake for ten to twelve minutes, and let cool before serving.

Keep in Mind:

Now you have everything at your disposal to control your diabetes. Remember that even though many of these things can help with type one diabetes, they are mainly meant to help you to control type two diabetes, which is a little easier to control and much more likely to be controlled without the use of medication. Of course, talk to your doctor before adding any supplements or herbs into your daily regime. Sticking to a proper diet and exercise will be the main key, and these recipes should help motivate you to do so and get you started.

Also, remember that everyone reacts differently to different recipes and their ingredients, so you need to still check your blood sugar levels to make sure a recipe is really right for you, and usually it's not a single recipe or a single meal that determines how well your blood sugar levels are for the day. Try to stay on an even keel by knowing what you can and cannot pair together in a single day.

www.ingramcontent.com/pod-product-compliance
Lightning Source LLC
Chambersburg PA
CBHW070031040426
42333CB00040B/1425